CALISTHENICS

THE ULTIMATE GUIDE TO BODYWEIGHT EXERCISE

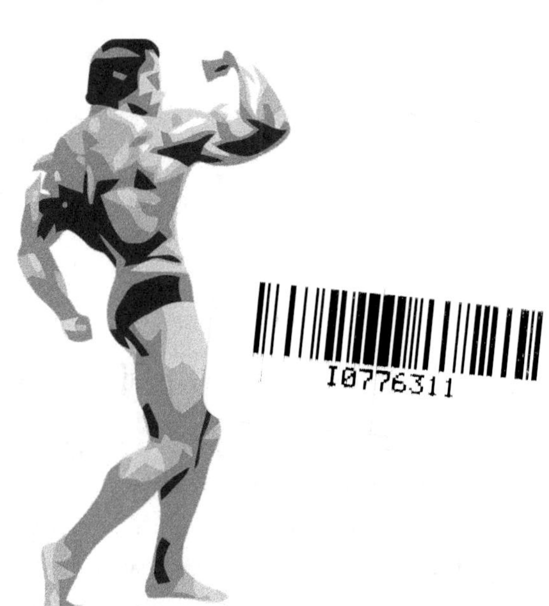

BONUS!!

Wouldent it be great to have new books sent to your email for **free**? Or even Keen up on some some tips an tricks with training ? How about some help with your diet?

Just click the link below an to receive your first of many *TIPs* on muscle building *SECRETS*

Just visit Http://eepurl.com/c-iwx1 to opt in

TABLE OF CONTENTS

INTRODUCTION

Calisthenics is fast becoming one of the most sought-after exercise programs that fitness professionals, coaches and trainers are incorporating into their fitness regimes to further enhance the effectiveness of their training program. What exactly is calisthenics?

Calisthenics basically consists of exercises that involve bodyweight only. It may involve the use of equipment, but this is not necessary. These exercises include, but not limited to, jumping, doing push-ups, swinging, chin-ups etc. All of these exercises have proven to increase flexibility, muscle coordination and agility.

Calisthenics is a form of strength and power training utilizing only compound bodyweight exercises. Training the muscles in isolation doesn't teach the body how to coordinate its strength and balance through the core – calisthenics helps you to develop that through the pursuit of clean and Strict Form. The techniques learned can then be mixed with each other into routines (Freestyle Calisthenics or Street Workout), or weight can be added to the movement once strict form has been achieved to keep overloading the body.

Calisthenics strengthens the body holistically as a unit – it is incredibly useful for those who use their bodies for performance, for example in sports, martial arts, dance and yoga. Whether you are aiming to improve your ability to keep possession of a ball, developing your punching or kicking power, perfecting your balance or simply just to get stronger, Calisthenics is an age old training system which will benefit you hugely.

There are many examples of calisthenics workout, which you can incorporate into your fitness training.

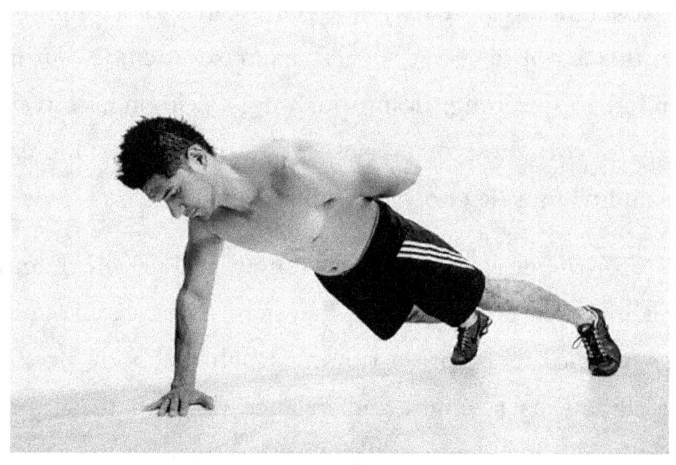

Chapter 1
Calisthenics

Getting Fit At Home without Weights

Exercises that involve equipment and weights are best done under the supervision of a trainer. Undoubtedly, with these gears, having a trained pro around can prevent a lot of exercise-related injuries. A fitness professional can also design a regimen to specifically suit your health and individual needs.

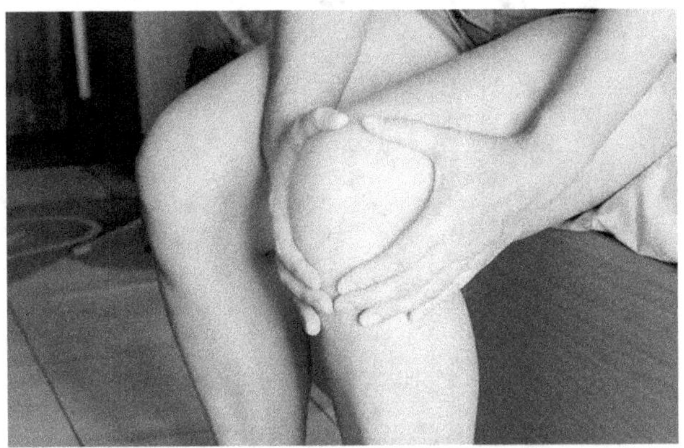

But not all of us have the time or energy to go to the gym or afford a personal trainer. But this does not mean that you can kiss working out goodbye. To keep fit, you have to work out. And yes, you can do your own home workout without the weights.

The answer is **Calisthenics**

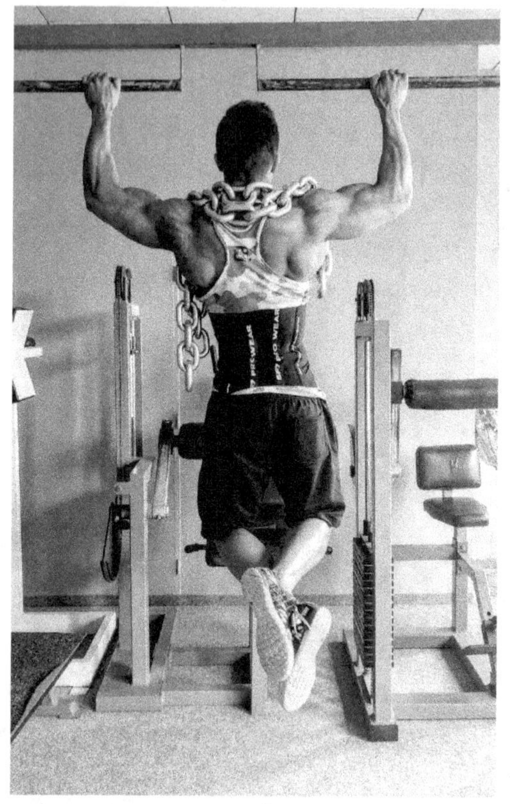

If this is the first time you've heard of calisthenics, read on. Calisthenics are dynamic exercises that are simple and rhythmical in nature. It's a form of bodyweight exercise that consists of bending, jumping, twisting and kicking that strengthens and builds muscle mass. Take note, however, that calisthenics won't give you the body of Arnold Schwarzenegger in his prime. It will, however, make your body more supple and give you that added boost of confidence.

Calisthenics is also an exercise that even hypertensive individuals can perform. Like any other exercise, calisthenics increases blood pressure but unlike high-impact exercises, there's no danger of getting it to reach uncontrollable levels. A regular calisthenics exercise lowers bad cholesterol while increasing the good kind. It enables the body to lose those excess pounds and consequently, improve your overall physical appearance.

In the beginning, a 10-minute calisthenics exercise would serve its purpose. As soon as you gain strength, stamina and the mental determination to do more, you can gradually increase your workout schedule. Push-ups, crunches, pull-ups, lunges, flutter kicks and squats are just some of the more common calisthenics exercises.

In doing push-ups, make sure that your arms go from fully extended in your starting position to almost fully flexed as you bend down low, making sure that you don't rest on the floor. Crunches are similar to sit-ups except you only tighten the abdominal muscles. Pull-ups are performed with an overhead bar (or a strong tree branch as an alternative). You lift your body up slowly while keeping your back straight until it reaches chin level and return to normal position also in a slow and tightly-controlled manner. Lunges are done by simply bringing the leg to a 90 degree angle in front of you with the other leg on a semi-kneeling position behind you. You then stand up and do the same to the other leg. Flutter kicks are done in a lying position, with your hands behind your buttocks as you move up your feet up and down close to the ground. Squats are done with feet and shoulders wide apart. You then squat as far down as possible while bringing your arms forward before resuming to a standing position.

So if you're looking for that safe and complete home workout that you can do every day minus the weights, calisthenics is your best bet. It doesn't only make you lose weight; it improves your posture and boosts your self-image, too. What more could you possibly want in a workout?

Calisthenics for Excellent Total Body Conditioning

If you want to talk about getting into superior shape then you have got to include calisthenics into your regular day to day workout regimen. Kalli-Sthenos is the Greek origin of the word calisthenics. Kalli (beautiful) sthenos (strength) is where the word calisthenics comes to life. So what are calisthenics? Well basically calisthenics involve whole body movements and exercises that are performed in a rhythmic and systematic way in order to promote muscular strength, mobility, and cardiovascular fitness all at once. This can be done with nothing more than your own body weight and will allow you to get a superior workout.

Total Body Conditioning

Calisthenics are great for anyone to perform in order to get into shape for any reason. The fact is that it doesn't matter if you are an athlete or regular fitness junkie you will benefit greatly from this form of physical training. The great thing about this form of training is that it can be done just about anywhere and at any time.

You see some examples of calisthenics involve drills such as jumping jacks, squat thrusts, and burpees. These exercises all have multiple steps and actions that must be understood and performed by the participant in a flowing manner in order to obtain there full benefits. You see smart training must involve the process of connecting the mind and body in harmony in order to be effective. If you are relying on the mindless bicep curl machine to get you fit then you will never get there. You can't function without both the mind and body working together towards executing a task. It's simply impossible.

Calisthenics are a great way for you to sharpen your skills in exercising. This particular form of training allows you to maintain an "edge" much like the blade of a knife would when used and sharpened regularly over time. If you don't use and sharpen the blade it will simply dull and rust resulting in complete uselessness. Here is an important message for you; your body will do the same thing if you don't use it properly! If you haven't already you have got to engage in fundamental fitness and strength with calisthenics.

CHAPTER 2
CALISTHENICS FOR MASS BUILDING

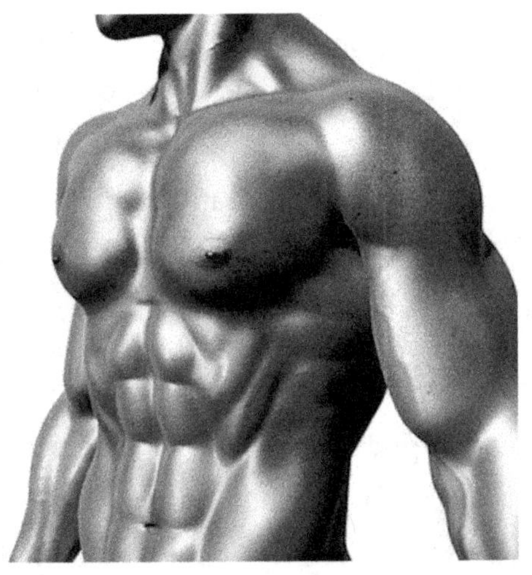

There is very little in this world which can escape the push and pull of changing trends - and muscle building workouts are no exception. For the last decade, gyms up and down the country have been filled with pumped up guys, worshiping at the altar of the bench press and the dumbbell rack.

Yet, what happens if you turn up for your session and there is a queue of hulking gents hogging the rack? What if you cannot make it to the gym at all? You might have to work away from home. You might have a hard month and have to cancel your membership outright. Are you supposed to just let all of those hard won gains go to waste?

Of course not - men built mass before the invention of sophisticated gym machines and they can still do it now. In fact, this more organic way of building muscle (commonly referred to as bodyweight training or calisthenics) has slowly grown in popularity over the last five years. There are now more guys choosing to trust their bodies and acquire mass the natural way.

Whilst weight training with apparatus is certainly not a bad way to sculpt and tone the chest, arms, and back, a narrow emphasis on assisted training often leads to a physicality which is overly reliant on a limited range of forms. Alternatively, calisthenics (or bodyweight training), which tones and shapes, via strength training without weights, encourages the body to become flexible, supple, incredibly strong under pressure.

Balanced Calisthenics for Sustainable Mass

The real power in calisthenics training lies with the fact that it focuses on movements which involve multiple muscles. It does not try to pick out and strengthen separate muscle groups. This is something which can feel rather alien to anybody who is unfamiliar with bodyweight exercises, but its value quickly becomes clear when trying to learn how to master tricky moves like the one arm pull up.

Clearly, a one arm pull up is going to require super strong arms and laterals, but it needs more than this. In fact, it cannot be done without the ability to regulate strength and tension across the whole of the body. This is what calisthenics does; it involves the whole body as a cohesive unit, order to create balanced and even centers of mass.

The core tenets of calisthenics strength training exhibit a direct physical expression, as the strength to weight balance needed to carry out high level exercises makes precise demands on the body. For this reason, calisthenics experts work towards finding the perfect balance between muscle mass and body fat, so that no cycle, movement, or exercise is beyond them.

Calisthenics for the Abs

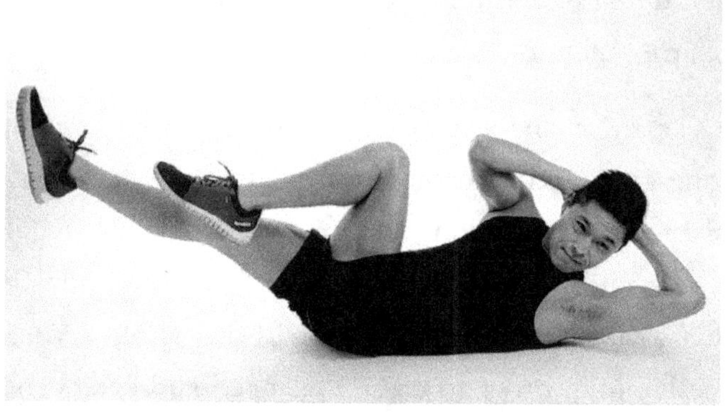

The best calisthenics 'projects' begin right at the center. This is important because, in order to use your own weight as a tool, you first need to train your abs to withstand the pressure - calisthenics routines always rely on the abs. It will start to show after a couple of months too, so keep that end goal in mind if the work feels intimidating.

The windshield wiper and the hanging leg raise are both great moves for working the abs. In fact, any kind of bar work is bound to be valuable. The classic bar move puts pressure on the serratus anterior, and it produces visible changes within the torso very quickly. If you want that killer serratus edge and a six pack to die for, this is the way to go.

Calisthenics for the Arms

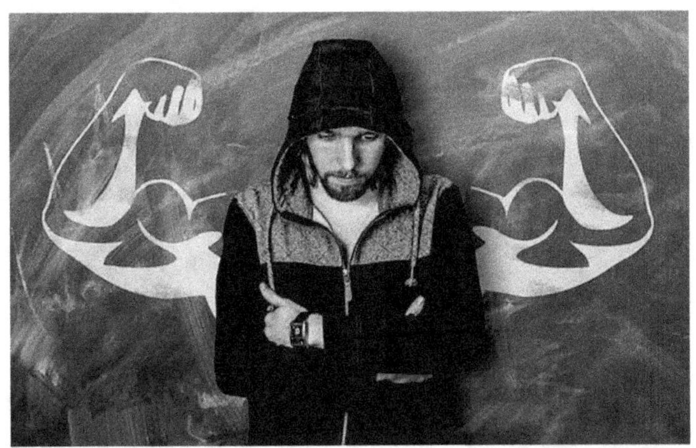

To start making gains in this area, you do not even have to switch up your moves all that much - bar work happens to be great for arms too, especially biceps. The truth is that your arms are going to get a more solid workout from chin up reps than they are curls, so keep using your own weight as tool and start worshiping the natural way.

There is a wide range of different moves that you could try here; everything from overhand pull ups to underhand chins, the thick bar, the switch grip, and pulling up from anything which is strong enough to take your weight. After a few months, you will start to notice an incredible increase in tensile capacity. You might start to look a bit like Popeye too, what with those arms.

Calisthenics for the Chest and Back

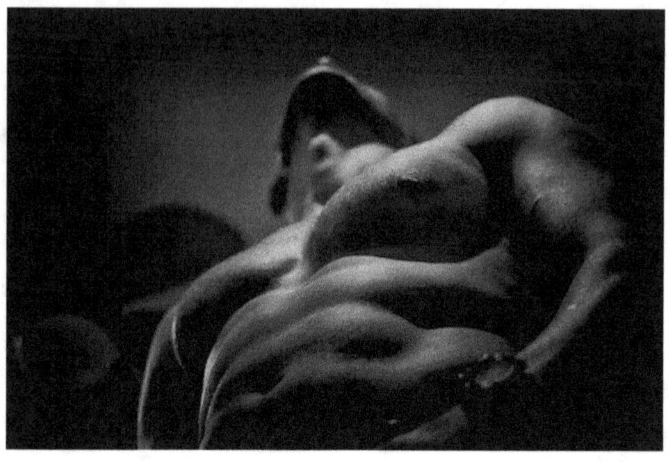

It should come as no surprise to find that extremely broad laterals are a real sign of an accomplished calisthenics built physique. As there is no narrow focus on picking out and separately working the arms, it becomes easier to realize the true potential of the laterals with the use of muscle ups, pull ups, bar levels, and moves like the human flag.

And now to the big boss of calisthenics; the classic push up. It remains one of the finest and most efficient unassisted bodyweight movements. However, too many guys are tempted to just get to grips with the boring old signature push up - take things further and make it exciting. You should always remember that if it is easy, your body is not working as hard as it should.

Putting Together the Right Calisthenics Routine

The following three day split calisthenics routine is a fairly basic one, but it will encourage the growth of new muscle. It can be performed with the use of exterior weights, or you can go solo and pump it out unassisted - the choice is yours.

Also, you can make the routine harder, if you need to, by altering the incline of push-ups, restricting points of contact, and expanding the range of motion, in order to definitively answer the question 'Can calisthenics build mass?'

Workout One: Pushing Movements + Core

- Exercise - Sets - Reps - Rest

- Weighted Push-up - 3 - 8-12 - 90 sec

- Weighted Push-up feet elevated - 3 - 8-12 - 90 sec

- Handstand Push-up - 3 - 8-12 - 90 sec

- Hanging Leg Raise - 3 - 12-15 - 90 sec

- Windshield Wipers - 3 - 12-15 - 90 sec

Workout Two: Pulling Movements + Core

- Exercise Sets Reps Rest

- Pull-up - 3 - 8-12 - 90 sec

- Neutral grip pull-up - 3 - 8-12 - 90 sec

- Chin-up - 3 - 8-12 - 90 sec

- Dragonflags - 3 - Failure - 180 sec

Workout Three: Legs and Conditioning:

- Exercise - Sets - Reps - Rest

- 100-meter Sprint - 3 - 150 sec

- 50 meter run, than 50 meter walk - 2 - 5 - 240 sec

- Pistol Squats - 3 - Pre-Fail - 150 sec.

- 7 Jump Squats

- 7 Jump Lunges (left)

- 7 Jump Lunges (right) - 3 - 90 sec.

Benefits of Calisthenics for Speed Training

Calisthenics are perfect for getting in proper shape for running and for gaining the break-neck speed you need to win trophies and make headlines. But some runners and speed training athletes feel that calisthenics aren't necessary for getting faster. And some are under the misconception that calisthenics training actually makes you slower. That couldn't be further from the truth. The following calisthenics benefits for speed training should clear the matter up nicely.

Introduces Variety into Your Training

One of the best benefits of engaging in calisthenics is the fact that you are getting tons of variety in your speed training workout. When you incorporate knee raises, pushups, crunches and planks with very few rests in between sets, you are conditioning your body to be as fast as possible. Remember to keep pushing yourself and to keep trying out different exercises so that you can condition your body even more.

Improves Coordination

When you speak of calisthenics benefits for speed training, you can't leave out coordination. Coordination plays a huge role when it comes to how fast you are, and if your coordination is off just a little bit you won't be able to increase your turnover rate and other runners will eventually blow right past you. But if you engage in various calisthenics a few times per week, you'll become much more coordinated and your speed will increase as a result.

You'll Get Stronger

One of the most obvious calisthenics benefits for speed training include the fact that you will be getting stronger with each session. Of course you'll need to make sure you're getting plenty of fuel in the form of healthy foods and beverages and that you're getting plenty of rest, but if you do calisthenics in the form of pushups and leg raises and all the other exercises you tend to do when you're training, you will get stronger and that will increase your power and, ultimately, your speed.

What Does It All Mean?

Hopefully by how you are convinced that you need calisthenics in your training regimen if you want to develop the kind of speed that makes others, including college scouts, take notice. You don't want to be the slowest person on the field and you certainly don't want to be second place. You want to win, and that's why you train every chance you get, using all the tools you've been taught in order to carry you towards your winning goals. But if you don't include calisthenics with the rest of your tools, you will eventually reach your glass ceiling and that's where you'll stay. So instead, realize the calisthenics benefits for speed training and train the way the experts do. Calisthenics are not 'old-school' or outdated, and they certainly won't make you any slower. Instead, they'll make you more coordinated, stronger and faster than ever. If you don't believe it, try incorporating calisthenics into your normal routine and you'll reach any speed-training goals you reach for yourself, guaranteed.

CHAPTER 3
ALL THAT YOU NEED TO KNOW ABOUT CALISTHENICS EXERCISES

Calisthenics is a form of workout where one uses only their body weight to achieve strength and get in shape. Calisthenics exercises can be practiced without much machinery or elaborate gym structures. The basic idea is to get endurance, stamina, flexibility and strength without depending on any tools or sophisticated equipment.

Calisthenics workouts are designed differently for everyone according to their fitness level and medical history. Without doubt it is one of the most suitable branches of fitness for those who like to enjoy wholesome health. It is this display of brawn and body control that has turned it into a sport that many people enjoy practicing and competing with.

The Fundamentals of Calisthenics Workout

Calisthenics is a versatile genre of workout where one's body weight is used as resistance. Equipment usage is kept to the minimum with basic tools like pull-up and dip bars, which can be bought from a local market or welded at home. Most people are drawn to it because these exercises can be performed almost anywhere. You can have some bars installed in your backyard and you are good to go.

Who Can Practice Calisthenics Exercises

Calisthenics is for everyone but as the form is based on body strength and endurance, it will need some getting used to with training and patience. People who are new to fitness and exercise routines may take up to six months to be able to perform all basic movements smoothly.

Calisthenics workout can be used to reach all kinds of health targets. Some athletes and bodybuilders practice them to increase power and body suppleness. The workout has various levels and so can be used to achieve all kinds of goals.

It is an ideal workout for weight loss, lean muscle build up, core strength and overall body coordination and shape.

Even if you do not have definite health goals and like to enjoy good health in general, calisthenics exercises will do the trick.

Types of Calisthenics Exercises

Calisthenics cannot be defined into a category as it involves anything and everything that promotes body-weight training. There are certain types of exercises, however, which can be done at the beginner's level. Once a person is adept at these, they can be incorporated into circuit training or other forms to reap better results.

Some examples of Calisthenics Workouts:

Planks: Planking helps your core and abs to gain strength.

Get into a prone position on the floor, supporting your weight on your toes and your forearms.

Keep your body straight all time, and hold this position as long as you can. To increase difficulty, an arm or leg can be raised.

Dips: Dips are a compound, body-weight exercise. They can do wonders for your upper body strength, working your chest, shoulders, back and arm muscles.

You do Dips by first raising yourself on two dip bars with straight arms. Lower your body until your shoulders is below your elbows. Push yourself up until your arms are straight again.

Squats: These are usually beneficial for legs and trains primarily the muscles of the thighs, hips and buttocks.

Stand with feet a little wider than shoulder-width apart, hips stacked over knees, and knees over ankles.

Keep the head facing forward with eyes straight ahead for a neutral spine. While the butt starts to stick out, make sure the back stays straight and the chest and shoulders stay upright.

Pull-ups: A pull-up is an upper-body compound pulling exercise. Chin pull ups and other varieties help build your back, arms, shoulders and strengthen your core.

Grab the pull-up bar with the palms facing forward or backward. Grip the bar shoulder-width apart with straight arms. Pull yourself up by pulling your elbows to the floor.

Keep pulling until your chin passes the bar. Lower yourself all the way down until your arms are straight, and then pull yourself up again.

Note on grips: For a wide grip, your hands need to be spaced out at a distance wider than your shoulder width. For a medium grip, your hands need to be spaced out at a distance equal to your shoulder width and for a close grip at a distance smaller than your shoulder width.

Pushups: A push-up is a common calisthenics exercise performed in a prone position by raising and lowering the body using the arms. Pushups are used to develop chest and triceps muscles. Get into a high plank position. Place your hands firmly on the ground; flatten your back so your entire body is neutral and straight.

Lower your body and Push back up. Keeping your core engaged exhale as you push back to the starting position.

Squat Thrust

These are a full body exercise which virtually works a lot of muscles in the body, from abs, glutes & hip flexors to chest and shoulders. You can burn more calories in a lot less time.

The start position is standing straight with your feet shoulder width apart and hands by your sides. Squat down and place your hands palms down on the floor in front of your feet. Jump your legs out behind you until they are fully extended, do 1 full push up and jump your feet forward to just behind your hands. Use an explosive motion to push through your heels and return to the start position.

Explosive Jumping Lunges

Targeting primary muscle groups: Quads and Hamstrings

Secondary: Abs, Calves, Glutes & Hip Flexors.

- Stand straight with a tight core and your chest up. Lunge forward with your right leg then put your hands on your hips and Jump up, switch your leg in midair, and land with your left leg in a forward lunge.

Alternate sides for one minute

Calf Raises

The standing calf raise exercise targets your calf muscles, particularly the larger, outermost muscle that is responsible for the shape and size of your calves. The muscles of the calf are viewed as an aesthetic priority more than anything else.

- Stand straight with a tight core and flat back.

- Keep your hands at your sides or hold on to a wall for balance.

- Bring your feet to be hip distance apart. Raise your heels by extending your ankles as high as possible and flexing your calf.

- Pause at the top and slowly return to the starting position.

Hanging Leg Raise

The hanging leg raise is a core strengthening exercise that targets the entire abdominal area and improves stability in the lower back and help strengthen other muscle groups such as your arms, shoulders and even your legs.

Grip a pull up bar with a firm overhand grip. Raise your legs until the torso makes a 90-degree angle, and then lower your legs slowly until they are straight and repeat.

Abs Exercises:

Abdominal area workouts help you get more control over your body movements besides giving you appealing six-pack abs.

There are several benefits associated with abs exercises. For example, it helps your body to attain a better posture because your muscles will be stronger. Also, those workouts will banish back pain and you'll notice that your lower back will be more flexible, and your digestion will improve through regular stomach exercise as well.

If you're starting an exercise routine to decrease your excess fat, it's important to focus on the lower abs first because this area is the most difficult to strengthen and tone. The upper abs will tone and tighten naturally as the lower abs become stronger. Calisthenics are a safe and result oriented form that really works.

CHAPTER 4
BASIC CALISTHENICS

Fitness Made To Order

Basic calisthenics, Well, if you're old enough to remember Physical Education Class (sadly, this is dying out these days), ever played a sport or been in the Military, you know exactly what I mean. Basic calisthenics are the exercise method of choice to build strong, conditioned bodies with little or no equipment.

Unfortunately, in today's world with expensive gyms full of shiny equipment and the fitness industry marketing "quick", "easy" fitness gimmicks, bodyweight calisthenics are often overlooked.

You would think bodyweight exercise would be the most widely used form of exercise because of its accessibility, versatility and effectiveness. After all, bodyweight calisthenics can be used by complete beginners all the way up to elite athletes to improve performance, heath and physique. But, many men and women have been convinced (brainwashed) that basic calisthenics pale in comparison to other forms of training.

Basic calisthenics should be the starting point for any physical training program, and should remain an integral part of your exercise program.

There is a place for calisthenics exercise in everyone's exercise program, ranging from being the full workout program to being a part of the over-all workout plan. Your body has always been, and will always be, the greatest tool for improving fitness, burning fat and building a strong, lean, athletic body. So, let's take a look at some of the ways you can start using basic calisthenics today!

Basic Calisthenics Make an Excellent Warm Up

Before you start any physical training, a proper warm up should be performed. And, in my opinion, there is no better warm up for every type of physical activity than bodyweight calisthenics. There is no other activity that can prepare your body for the multitude of movements of sport, work and life quite like bodyweight exercise.

Basic Calisthenics Make a Great Full Body Workout

You can use bodyweight exercise to improve upper body, lower body and core strength and endurance. Plus, the rhythmic nature of some calisthenics makes them excellent heart and lung workouts. So you can get a true full body workout which includes all muscle groups and the cardiorespiratory systems. And the best part, you don't need any equipment!

Mix Bodyweight Exercises with Other Forms of Training

Just because you use some other form of training, like dumbbells, barbells and machines, doesn't mean you shouldn't mix in some calisthenics as well. Just think about it. The challenges of sport, work and life require moving the weight of your own body, moving other objects or moving your own bodyweight and other objects. You should train accordingly by mixing bodyweight exercise and weighted resistance.

You Can Do Bodyweight Cardio Intervals

At the end of most people's workout, they do some "cardio". Unfortunately, this often means zoning out on the treadmill or exercise bike while reading a magazine or watching the T.V. It is suggested that you pump up the intensity by throwing in some Bodyweight Intervals. Every once in a while, jump off the bike or treadmill and do some basic calisthenics. This boosts the intensity of your workout by breaking your breathing and heart rhythms, ultimately providing a better workout.

Effective Benefits of Bodyweight Training

The words workout or exercise may not induce a happy reaction in you, but let me tell you about some really great benefits that show just how great calisthenics exercises are for your body and mind.

Some of the benefits of calisthenics workouts that everybody talks about are:

- Calisthenics Workouts will give you more energy and improve the quality of sleep. When you are working up you will find that you do not need to sleep as much and you will have more energy to complete your training.

- Calisthenics workouts decrease depression. Regular calisthenics are an excellent way to boost your mood, regulate your emotions and get in shape. When you exercise, your body releases endorphins, adrenaline, serotonin and dopamine. These are the body's natural feel good chemicals. They work together to make you feel good. Try to train three days a week for about 45 minutes and your body will thank you.

- When you do calisthenics, you burn calories. So, when you want to go and have your favorite ice-cream, if you do your exercises that ice cream will not land on your waistline, thighs or hips, which is where fat generally goes. The visual result of calisthenics workouts is that you will burn fat and gain lean muscles at the same time.

- All calisthenics exercises are something that you can learn easily, on your own and that you will be able to do in your own home. All that you need is your body weight, the ground and the earth's gravity. You do not have to buy five hundred dollars weight equipment or get a gym membership. What you need is an affordable training guide, a manual that will teach you the proper form and technique on every bodyweight exercise so you will start your great physical transformation.

- These bodyweight exercises are ideal for both beginners as well as those with more experience who wish to push or test the limits of their strength, endurance or physical capabilities.

- Calisthenics are the only training workout that will sculpt your body the natural way.

These are some of the most talked about benefits of calisthenics workouts.

In all honesty, calisthenics exercise is great because it allows you to feel good about yourself, feel good about your body.

But, you see, there are a million different other benefits with calisthenics: it reduces the risk of cancer, it reduces cholesterol, it reduces the risk for diabetes, it reduces your body fat, it increases metabolism, and it enhances flexibility, agility, coordination and range of motion. It improves digestion, it decreases dramatically the negative effects of ageing, it increase self-awareness and life span, it increases bone density, it improves brain function and reflexes.

The bottom line is that Calisthenics Workouts are worth the effort for life.

Are Basic Calisthenics Better Than Gym Machines?

When it's time to improve fitness, burn off ugly fat and build muscle, most men and women think of going to the gym and using gym machines. They completely skip over the power of basic calisthenics to build the strong, lean, muscular body they seek. This is a big mistake, and this article will show you why.

What Do We Mean By Basic Calisthenics?

When we say basic calisthenics we are talking about the bodyweight exercises you probably learned as a kid in gym class. Or, if you've ever seen a military movie, it is the calisthenics exercises the soldiers did in boot camp.

Some of the most well-known are jumping jacks, push-ups, bodyweight squats, squat thrusts and crunches... but there are hundreds of others and variations. These movements use only the weight of your own body as resistance, and train the body to move better in the way your body naturally moves. Bodyweight calisthenics are a great way to strengthen the entire body, improve heart and lung power and burn off fat.

Why people who do Calisthenics workouts don't Like Gym Machines

When you join a gym, they usually don't spend too much time on basic calisthenics. (After all, why teach you to do something effective at building the body you want without needing a gym). They strap you into shiny gym machines with seat belts and have you do a wide variety of movements. Unfortunately, these movements are often foreign to the way your body moves.

One of the biggest reasons they don't like gym machines is because of the Principle of Specificity.

Basically, your body makes adaptations due to the specific stresses placed upon it. This means your body becomes better at performing gym machine exercises.

But didn't you join the gym to improve your performance, health and appearance OUTSIDE the gym?

Why Basic Calisthenics Are Better Than Gym Machines

There are obvious reasons some prefer bodyweight calisthenics over gym workouts. You can do them anywhere, anytime. You don't need an expensive gym membership or costly equipment. And they work!

But the biggest reason I like bodyweight workouts better is they train the body to perform better in ways that are applicable to your work, sport and life activities. Unless you get strapped into machines in your real life, bodyweight calisthenics produce better results!

The next time you look in the mirror and decide it's time to get into shape, burn fat or build a more athletic looking body, don't immediately grab your credit card and head off to the local gym. You already have the best gym in the world... your own body. All you have to do is learn to use it.

The best three key ways to achieve your Calisthenics workout goals

There are a thousand training programs, pills and diets that are supposed to help you with your health and fitness. Some of them really help and inspire people, but some will cheat you with short-term results that do not lead to best long-term health and fitness.

Keep in mind that when it comes to calisthenics workouts, the winning approach must incorporate your motivation, your training and your nutrition. We are going to show you an overview of those three keys ways to achieve your long-term fitness and health goals.

Motivation

Let's start with motivation. With motivation, we can look at your philosophy, your attitude and your goals. Obviously, goals are very important. You must first set a goal in order to achieve one. The benefits of bodyweight calisthenics workouts are so obvious that it seems impossible to forget them and yet sometimes we do. We let things get in the way. We let other priorities overtake our own health and fitness. Yet, our health and fitness is the one area of our life that has a positive effect on all other arias.

It is important that when you are setting your goals, you must touch some powerful reasons for having those goals. For example, I want to lose ten pounds so that I feel great about myself or I want to run two miles so that I can keep up with my children and be a good parent. Set your goals, but do not forget to set some powerful reasons for having those goals. This is the only way to keep your level of motivation high, in your everyday life.

Also with motivation, you need to look at your attitude and philosophy. Attitude is the precursor for what you do. If you do not have a good attitude, you likely will not have good actions. For instance, if you are thinking that you do not have time to do your calisthenics workouts, you are wrong. You have a bad attitude and your priorities are mixed up. You need to change your attitude before you will ever change.

If you are not doing the right things and you are not getting the rights results, you need to look at what you are thinking. Here is the issue; you control your thoughts not the other way around. You need to take control and your philosophy will help you do it.

Philosophy takes the attitude to a deeper level. You can choose your philosophy and you can choose what you accept to be. For example, you have a philosophy in your life that calisthenics workouts are a necessity for the duties and the pleasures.

You must look at your philosophy, your attitude and your goals in approaching your health and fitness goals.

Training

The second important key is training. The best calisthenics workouts involve three aspects: resistance bodyweight training, cardiovascular bodyweight training and flexibility training.

Resistance calisthenics workouts include bodyweight exercises and they are vital for maintaining and increasing your muscle tone and your strength.

Cardiovascular calisthenics training incorporates cardiovascular bodyweight fitness and it is great for burning body fat.

Flexibility training will protect you from injuries. It will help you maintain good posture and good movement in all of your joins.

Nutrition

The third important key is nutrition. There is so much information out there that you don't know what to accept. However, you do not want to go on a diet, which is a short-term fix. You want to teach yourself about nutrition and learn the correct principles of healthy eating.

If you can put your motivation, your training and your nutrition together, there is a guarantee you that you will enjoy better health, fitness and life.

Calisthenics Workouts - The Proper Hydration

Although calisthenics workouts are the best way to burn fat and gain muscle at the same time, calisthenics nutrition is an important step on the road to successful training.

But, pay attention. Calisthenics nutrition is not all about food. Getting enough to drink is also a key part of your fitness success. Proper hydration is very important in your everyday life, let alone during the intense calisthenics workouts.

The funny thing about proper hydration is that everybody is telling us what to drink instead of what not to. Therefore, we are going to mention four of the worst possible things that you can drink: alcohol, diet drinks, coffee and non-organic milk.

Alcohol: Excessive alcohol promotes dehydration and depletes your B vitamins and magnesium, which are essential for progesterone. The people who drink excessively in the long run develop cirrhosis of the liver. Bottom line: alcohol is bad. Limit it as much as possible.

Diet and Sport Drinks: These highly publicized drinks contain a large amount of artificial sweeteners that promote your body's cravings for real sugar. Artificial sweeteners will change your metabolic process and you will be tempted to eat and drink more sugar-based products. You will have the tendency to gain weight instead of losing it. And you do not want that, do you? Another big problem with the diet and sport drinks is they are loaded with caffeine. As you know by now, caffeine is responsible for dehydration, headaches and hallucinations for heavy users of diet and energy drinks.

Coffee: Do not get me wrong, a cup of coffee is good for you! Sugar free coffee is good because it speeds up fat metabolism during calisthenics workouts and it increase intellectual activity. It has five times the anti-oxidants of the green tea. It is an excellent anti-depressant and it enhances performance and memory. Coffee also has a very protective effect against cirrhosis of the liver and against prostate or colon cancer. However, you should not drink coffee if you get agitated or if you have high blood pressure. It is also recommend to be drinking organic coffee, as inorganic is sprayed with dangerous pesticides. Moderation is the key.

Non-organic milk: Although milk is rich in essential nutrients, in calcium and other alkaline minerals, non-organic milk is far from healthy. The calves are fed with genetically modified food. Unfortunately, there are not a whole lot of studies that are showing the long-term side effects of genetically modified food. Dairy cows are pumped full of artificial growth hormones, steroids and antibiotics, which end up in the milk you drink. It is scientifically proven that these dangerous chemical substances will dramatically affect all your metabolic process. Organic milk is different. It is higher in omega 3 fatty acids. It is also much higher in vitamins and anti-oxidants than non-organic milk. I am sure many people will say that cow's milk is allergenic and this is true. The solution is to replace it with goat milk or vegetable milk (soy, oat or rice).

We may also add to the list of worst drinks the frozen mocha and hot chocolate, fruit juices from concentrate, soft drinks, ice cream sodas, frozen fruit drinks and drive-through shakes. Although considered bad beverages, all of these drinks can be consumed in moderation without having a significant impact on your calisthenics workouts or your health.

Keep in mind that your body needs water when you are thirsty, so water is the best drink ever.

CHAPTER 5
HOW TO DO A CALISTHENICS WORKOUT BETTER

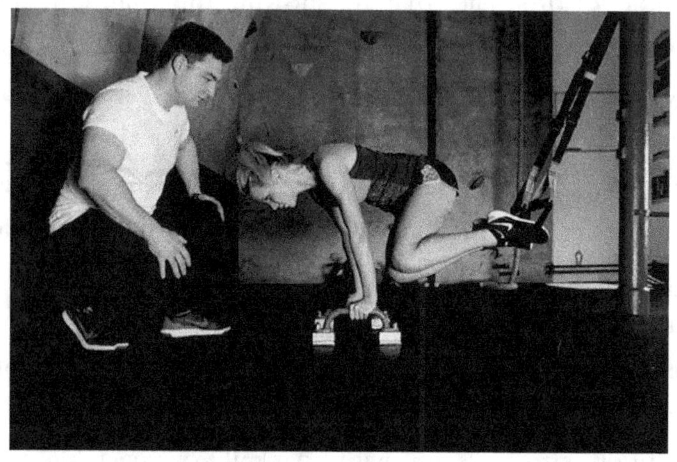

For some reason, people spend more time figuring out how to get the results they want with weight training than with a calisthenics workout. Weight lifters come up with complex calculations of weight, sets, reps, rest periods, nutrition etc. to gain an edge on getting superior results faster. But when it comes to bodyweight workouts, it seems like the one size fits all method rules.

It's like this stems from the mentality that bodyweight exercises are only good for moderate improvements and general fitness. And since it is believed to be a "mediocre" training method, it is only given "mediocre" attention.

This is a big mistake, and we are going to show you why you should strive to make your bodyweight workouts the best they can be.

Don't Rely On a One Size Fits All Calisthenics Program

You'll commonly see calisthenics used as a warm up for other forms of resistance training (weight lifting) or to improve general fitness. Basic bodyweight exercise like push-ups, crunches and squats come to mind. But this doesn't even scratch the surface of the power of bodyweight workouts.

Here is the truth. Bodyweight calisthenics can be just as effective as weight training to improve performance, burn off fat and build a muscular body. Therefore, just as much care and planning should be used to design your bodyweight only workout program as you would a weight training program. A one size fits all, "mediocre" workout program just won't do.

Use Multiple Calisthenics Workouts to Reach Your Ultimate Goal

Basically, there are three types of calisthenics workouts you should design. One targeted to general fitness, one to fat loss and one to strength and size. Why these three focuses? Because these are the three areas most people need to work on in order to reach their fitness, fat loss and physique goals.

In the weight lifting world workouts are often split up along these lines. And they should also be used in a bodyweight only program. The trick is to design the programs so they focus on a specific goal, without neglecting all other goals.

Blur the Lines between Strength Training and Cardio Conditioning

The biggest mistake both bodyweight exercisers and weight lifters do is insisting on splitting up their resistance training and cardio training. They divide their training so much that they don't get the best benefits.

In the real world, activities require the combined effort of all the muscles in your body, heart and lung power and mental toughness. Activities must be performed in a fluid manner switching between all three. You must blur the lines between your resistance training and cardio training.

Bodyweight calisthenics workouts make this easy. By using bodyweight exercises combined with fast paced calisthenics exercises, you can get a great workout that results in more real world benefits. If you want your body to respond in the face of real sport, work and life challenges, you must train it properly by challenging the entire body as one complete unit.

A calisthenics exercise program should be planned just as carefully as any other type of physical training. Design different workouts with different goals in mind. And push the limits by combining your resistance training and cardio training. You'll be happy with the results.

Calisthenics Routine - How to Prevent Getting Bored and Maximize Results

One of the biggest complaints people have about a calisthenics routine is that it is boring. The fact is that, if you do the same exercises over and again anyone would be bored to tears. Plus, doing the same bodyweight workout (or any workout for that matter), over and over is not the best way to keep the physical improvements coming. We are going to show you three ways to keep you from getting bored doing your bodyweight workouts and dramatically improve their effectiveness at the same time.

Use a Wide Variety of Bodyweight Exercises

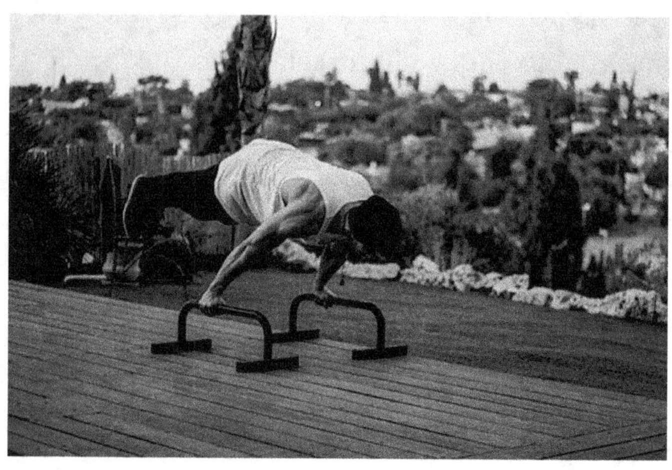

Frankly, there are so many different bodyweight exercises to use when designing your calisthenics routine, how could you possible get bored? There are hundreds of bodyweight exercises and calisthenics exercises to choose from. Plus there are countless ways to combine them into a great full body workout.

Sadly, most people only use a handful of bodyweight exercises. Keep from getting bored by learning and combining new exercises. This will also challenge your body in different ways and keep the physical improvements coming.

Use Different Bodyweight Workouts Focused On Different Results

Exercisers have different goals. So want to get fit. Some are more interested in burning fat. And others want to build attractive muscle for both performance and appearance. And the fact is a calisthenics routine is a great choice for each of these goals.

But there is not one best workout to achieve all these different goals. And what's worse, most people need to focus on ALL THREE to get the results they want. So, what do you do?

Use three different bodyweight calisthenics routines and rotate between them! Changing your workout focus from time to time keeps you on the path of progress toward your best body and keeps you from getting bored.

Combine Your Full Body Workout with Your Cardio Training

Exercisers like to know exactly why they are performing certain exercises. They like to know the exact muscles each exercise works. They want to know if the exercise is for strength, size, endurance, etc. This is why most people gravitate to bodybuilding style workouts followed by separate cardio workouts.

But I will say a more effective way to train is to attack your full body on all levels at the same time. Workout all the muscles in your body, your heart and lungs and test your mental toughness all at the same time.

You'll find that this type of combined training is more fun, more challenging and ultimately more effective at reaching your fitness, fat loss and physique building goals.

Look, if you want to get the most from your calisthenics routine there is no secret. You must do your bodyweight workouts consistently to get the results you seek. This means you cannot get bored and give up!

Use the three techniques mentioned above to keep your bodyweight calisthenics training interesting and more effective!

Guidelines for a Safe, Effective and Rewarding Bodyweight Calisthenics Program

Most people are familiar with some sort of bodyweight calisthenics program or another whether it is from gym class or a sport you were involved in. However, most people mistakenly think a bodyweight calisthenics program is "easy"... and often put themselves at risk.

Yes, you can still hurt yourself even when only using your own bodyweight as resistance.

A bodyweight calisthenics program is extremely safe, effective and rewarding if you follow some simple guidelines.

Guidelines for a Successful Bodyweight Calisthenics Program

Start Slow

Whether you are just starting a bodyweight calisthenics program, or including a bodyweight calisthenics program into current physical training... don't over-do it in the beginning.

Bodyweight calisthenics training is different than other forms of training, (leading to its effectiveness), and will stress the body in different manners than other forms of training, like weight lifting.

Don't underestimate bodyweight calisthenics exercises.

Warm Up Before and Cool Down After

A correctly planned bodyweight calisthenics program can be surprisingly challenging... and should be treated like other forms of strenuous exercise. A proper warm up and cool down is absolutely necessary.

You must prepare your body for the challenging exercise to come, and begin the repair process after physical activity.

Perform the Exercises Properly

Many people think they know how to perform the exercises making up their bodyweight calisthenics program properly but they don't! Bodyweight calisthenics exercise is one of the safest and most effective and rewarding form of exercise there is... if done properly!

Use a detailed guide with descriptions and photos to ensure proper performance of the exercises... and greatly reduce the risk of injury.

Think quality over quantity when performing your bodyweight calisthenics program.

Progress at Your Own Pace

In order to reap the rewards and benefits of your bodyweight calisthenics program... your training must be progressive. After all, if you're not improving over time, what's the point of training?

Unfortunately, most people limit themselves to one type of progression when using bodyweight calisthenics exercises... increasing reps. To get the most out of your bodyweight calisthenics program, and avoid overuse injuries... progress in multiple ways.

If you progress step-by-step on multiple levels, at your own pace... you will ensure every workout produces the best results for YOU.

In conclusion, A bodyweight calisthenics program is an excellent way to get in shape without costly equipment or expensive gym memberships, and is the most versatile and accessible physical training methods at your disposal. Treat your bodyweight calisthenics program with respect!

Don't let the "simple" nature of bodyweight calisthenics exercise fool you. Your bodyweight calisthenics program should be treated with the same safety and care as other forms of physical training.

Properly done, a bodyweight calisthenics program can be a stand-alone exercise program for fitness, health and physique... or an excellent addition to other forms of exercise.

Follow the above guidelines and enjoy the power of a safe, effective and rewarding bodyweight calisthenics program.

CHAPTER 6
HOW TO BUILD MORE MUSCLE

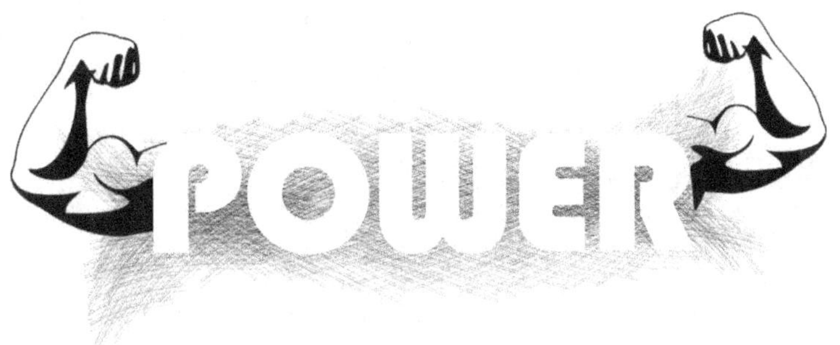

Building muscle has become a craze for many young men and women across the world. Those that are new to the sport of weightlifting or bodybuilding seek out body building routines in hopes to find better, quicker and perhaps easier way to build more muscle. This chapter will offer tips and guidance as to what you can do to achieve your muscle building goals.

You are probably already aware that several factors impact a person's ability to build more muscle. These include your own strength, consistency of working out, your eating habits and nutrition. All of these things combined will determine how efficiently you can develop lean muscle mass.

Never underestimate the power of nutrition in your training program. It is easy to think that all you have to do is lift weights and do some cardio to develop the physique that you want. If you aren't feeding your body the right kinds of nutrients then you will be spinning your wheels. I mean you wouldn't put a low grade fuel in a high performance race car, would you? Same with your body, if you want to get bigger and stronger, leaner and ripped you need to fuel your body with well-balanced foods and nutrients throughout the day.

If you are just starting out you probably are reading the muscles mags that outline what the professional bodybuilders are doing. That's not the worst thing you could do but don't think you should follow everything you read in those magazines. Don't try to keep up with their workouts. There are a lot of things that go on "behind the scenes" that we're not aware of. The models in the magazines are IFBB pros for a reason. That's not what we are. You can use those magazines for inspiration every now and then and at times to get a fresh idea on an old exercise. Never try to duplicate entire workout regimens.

Another important factor when choosing a body building routine and in wanting to build more muscle is to learn to go at your own pace. You may have role models and body builders that you want to emulate but everyone is different. Your body will respond differently to your workouts and you have to listen to what it is telling you. It's great to push yourself but if you feel like you need to rest or hold back then you'd better listen. This will help you reduce your risk of injury and prevent burnout.

Bodyweight Training - The Favored Training Method of Smart Body Builders

People who feel that a superb body can be achieved only by getting actively involved in a grueling gym schedule on a regular basis, can now take a look at bodyweight training exercises for a change! Yes, the same brilliant body shaping result that gym exercises offer you can now be accomplished from the comforts of your home. This is a machine-free mode of training which turns your body into your gym and guides it to provide the resistance and strength needed to make your exercises as effective as gym workouts.

Bodyweight training is the favored training method for many hard core body builders simply because of the conveniences and grand results that it offers in its most basic form. Anyplace - your home, office cubicle or rest room - can be the perfect place for bodyweight training exercises. Since it involves no equipments, it is also the cheapest and the most affordable method of working out. Because of its back-to-basics exercises, trainers always recommend this pattern of training to beginners who are starting fresh on body building schedules. Although intense and advanced exercises are a part of advanced bodyweight training, newcomers can start with the most simple squats and push-ups before progressing to advanced levels. Bodyweight exercises are a real fun way to blend different modes of training targeting different body zones, ultimately aiming to reach a total body strengthening workout result. A variety of bodyweight exercises are available for adoption like the handstand push-up, pull-up, inverted row, squat, split, calf raise, burpees, Mountain climbers and Boot Strappers. Any bodyweight training session can be the most effective when the best combination of exercises are ideally customized and combined as per individual comfort level, capacity and requirements. To tone the body from multiple dimensions must ideally be the primary goal for every trainer.

A bodyweight training schedule is the preferred choice of body builders worldwide as it is perfectly effective to spare you two hours of exhausting gym schedule every day and can still produce the best results when muscle building or fat burning is targeted. The workout regimen must be gradually built up in intensity and can be modified to fit the training pattern of newcomers, sedentary lifestyle people, active body building trainees, and advanced exercisers.

The initial bodyweight training phase concentrates on building up muscle endurance in the abs, lower back and upper body through general bodyweight low scale exercises which focus on strength training and body conditioning. In the next phase, bodyweight circuits are performed which can make you do some high calorie burning workouts of short time bouts. As your body gets stronger, the following phases target to build more muscle strength through advanced exercise plans. Since bodyweight training sessions are targeted to condition the whole body in parts and as a comprehensive whole, some advanced lower body strength building exercises are incorporated into the training regimen along with upper body conditioning exercises. These exercises may be without machines but be ready to get amazed at the difficulty levels of the single leg exercises of the lower body and the pushes and pulls that accompany it. Strength training and circuit conditioning work hand in hand in all phases of bodyweight training to bring you a leaner, stronger and powerful physique that is the dream of every body builder.

Do remember that guided bodyweight training is always better and is guaranteed to yield the desired results in the shortest possible time. Browse the net for the perfect training schedule that comes with the right amount of exercise information, videos and nutritional advice, so that you reach your body building and toning goal in the shortest possible time.